Fake Healing Claims
for HIV and AIDS

Copyright 2016 Klaus Fiedler

All rights reserved. No part of this publication may be reproduced, stored in a retrieval system, or transmitted in any form or by any means, electronic, mechanical, photocopying, recording or otherwise, without prior permission from the publishers.

Copying for non-commercial purposes is permitted within Malawi

Published by
Mzuni Press
P/Bag 201
Luwinga, Mzuzu 2
Malawi

ISBN 978-99960-45-26-4

Mzuni Press is represented outside Malawi by:

African Books Collective Oxford (also for e-books)
(orders@africanbookscollective.com)

www.mzunipress.blogspot.com

www.africanbookscollective.com

Printed in Malawi by Baptist Publications, P.O. Box 444, Lilongwe

Fake Healing Claims for HIV and Aids in Malawi: Traditional, Christian and Scientific

Klaus Fiedler

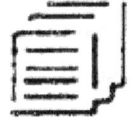
Mzuni Press

Mzuni Texts no. 5
2016

Contents

1. Introduction	6
1.1 Definition of healing	8
1.2 The areas treated in this book	10
2. Traditional healing claims	11
2.1 Chisupe	11
2.1.1 My sources	11
2.1.2 The events	12
2.1.3 The claims	13
2.1.4 The source of healing	13
2.1.5 The success	14
2.1.6 The false truth	14
2.1.7 Interpretations	15
2.2 Sing'anga	16
3. Chambe: "Healing the Nations"	17
4. A comparison: mixed agency healing claims outside Malawi	19
4.1. A herbal medicine from Tanzania and Congo	19
4.2. Rev Ambilikile Mwasapile, Tanzania	19
4.3 Prophet Stephen Kwagala, Uganda	20
5. Recent variants of multiple cure herbal drugs in Malawi	20
5.1 Teras!! The Wonderful Drug	20
5.2 Gloria Jeremiah's Herbal Hospital	21
5.3 The Hospital of Creation (Chipatala cha Chilengedwe)	22
5.4 Wizika	23
5.5 The false truth about herbs healing HIV/AIDS	24
6. Faith Healing HIV/AIDS	24
6.1 The false truth	24
6.2 Some observations	26
6.3 Nahori Malisa's research	27
6.3.1 Healed to death	28
6.3.2 A newspaper report	29
6.3.3 An assessment	29
6.4 Herbal HIV/AIDS medicine is less dangerous, but still...	31
6.5 The true truth about faith healing	33

6.6 What about ARVs?	34
6.6.1 The sin of pride	35
6.6.2 The witchcraft connection	35
7. The Voluntary Male Medical Circumcision Campaign	36
7.1 The false truth of VMMCC	37
7.2 The international origin of the campaign in Malawi	37
7.2.1 VMMCC as an additional method of reducing HIV transmission	39
7.2.2 Statistical evidence	39
7.4 The effects on women	41
7.5 The invisible condom or: The listener decides on the meaning of a message	42
7.5.1 A student's findings	43
7.6.1 Malawi Interfaith Association	45
7.6.2 Adventist Development Relief Agency (ADRA)	46
7.7 The Morality of the Voluntary Male Medical Circumcision Campaign	46
8. Conclusion	47
Bibliography	48
Unpublished	48
Published	48
Web	50

Note: Where appropriate names have been changed

1. Introduction

As far as human memory and archeological evidence go back, illness and death have been part of the human condition, and equally, as far back as human memory can reach, mankind has invested material and spiritual energies into delaying death by regularly treating and sometimes healing the illness that could bring about death. Much has been achieved, average life expectancy in better to do societies has probably doubled over the last centuries,[1] but, of course, death as the final reality of life has never been defeated.

As far as memory goes back, healing (or at least the attempt to heal) has been a human and as such a religious concern. In many traditional religions the healer is in the centre: In Celtic religion we find the Druid, the religions of Siberia are centred on the Shaman,[2] and it has been said that the most important religious official of African Traditional Religion, at least in Eastern and Central Africa, is the traditional doctor (*mganga, sing'anga, inyanga* etc). In all these forms of Traditional Religion healing has three components: biomedical, social and spiritual.

The biomedical side is primarily represented by herbal and other plant medicine,[3] but minerals can also be used or steam baths (among the Native Americans) or ablutions. The social side is included in the wholistic approach of not only looking at the illness of the body, but also at the sick social relationships of any patient.[4] Often traditional healing has strong spiritual components: Illness may come from God, and then there is no healing; illness may also have been caused by the breaking of a taboo, and in such a case neither herbs nor Western medicines will

---

[1] During my lifetime, my *statistical* life expectancy has grown by 7 years, for Germans.

[2] Nowadays the term is also applied to the Medicine Men (and Women) of the "Red Indians," now better called Native Americans.

[3] Chikanga, the famous witch finder, also used plants to treat different illnesses (Boston Soko, *Nchimi Chikanga. The Battle against Witchcraft in Malawi*, Blantyre: CLAIM-Kachere, 2002, pp. 52.)

[4] Depending on the approach used, this wholistic approach can be healing or destructive, as social tensions are often expressed in witchcraft fears and accusations. If the wholistic treatment protects "against the witches", it may well be healing, if the witch is named, however, the same wholistic approach magnifies the social tensions and is not healing but destructive.

help,[5] but going through the right ritual steps[6] or taking a specific medicine.[7] In other cases illness is seen as the consequence of neglect or an offence against an ancestor, then only an apology to and reconciliation with the offended ancestor will bring healing.[8] Probably the most frequent spiritual aspect of illness is that witchcraft is seen as the cause of a specific illness, so that fortification against witchcraft is required,[9] or purification from (conscious or sub-conscious) innate witchcraft[10] or naming and punishing the offender.[11] In traditional healing, wholistic as it is, there is no clear demarcation between spiritual, social and biomedical treatment and healing.

---

[5] A case here is *kanyera*, a deadly illness a man can contract when his penis touches his wife's menstrual blood. "Chinyela, chinyela, chitha amuna, Akazi atsala" (Rachel NyaGondwe Fiedler, *Coming of Age. A Christianized Initiation among Women in Southern Malawi*, Zomba: Kachere, 2005, p. 86). [*Chinyela* is the Yawo form of *Kanyera*].

[6] In the case of a breach of a *mdulo* taboo, the man who broke the taboo must arrange for another man to have sex with his wife before he, as her husband, can sleep with her again (Joseph DeGabriele, Joseph, "When Pills don't Work – African Illnesses, Misfortune and Mdulo," *Religion in Malawi*, No. 9, 1999, pp. 9-23).

[7] This is said to be a possible cure for *kanyera*, but only if taken very soon after the breach of the taboo (touching the wife's menstrual blood). I have not been able to find any details on that medicine.

[8] For detailed examples see: Joyce Mlenga, *Dual Religiosity in Northern Malawi*, Mzuzu: Mzuni Press, 2016, pp. 19f; 136.

[9] For this see ibid. p. 159.

[10] This was the major medical treatment administered by Nchimi Chikanga (Boston Soko, *Nchimi Chikanga. The Battle against Witchcraft in Malawi*, Blantyre: CLAIM-Kachere, 2002) and it is also a general pattern in all witchcraft eradication movements.

[11] This may increase tensions in the extended family or lead to social ostracism or expulsion from the village (especially if the accused are widows who still control a piece of land). Around the turn of the 19th to the 20th century the *mvabvi* oracle was frequently applied to exert such punishment.

1.1 Definition of healing

In this book I intend to relate these three forms of treatment and healing to one of the most difficult illnesses of our time, HIV/Aids. Before I can do that I need to define "healing". I see four levels:

(1) A cure that overcomes an illness and produces lifelong immunity against the same illness. Bubonic plague, measles and chicken pox are examples here.

(2) A cure that overcomes an illness, but where a recurrence of the same illness is possible. Here malaria, tuberculosis and stomach ulcers are examples.

(3) There are illnesses that are incurable, but that can be controlled by medicine.[12] Since the illness remains present, there is, technically, no healing, but since the treatment has achieved much, it is a form of healing on the *practical* level.

(4) Limited healing ("alleviation"): The illness is still incurable, and medicine can not control it. This means there is no healing on either the fundamental or the practical level, but through medical treatment there is a substantial reduction of suffering.[13]

The first two levels are real ("full") healing, level (3) is practical healing and level (4) is no healing, but a worthwhile achievement of medical treatment.

As far as healing is concerned, I follow the Roman Catholic position that healing must be proven, not just claimed or pronounced. This requires time (for cancer medical professionals tend to rate a 5 year "remission"

---

[12] High blood pressure, commonly known as BP, belongs to this category. It is in most cases incurable (unless when it is a mere symptom of another illness) and, usually after quite some time, may cause the (sudden) death of the patient. While this is true, a tablet a day can in most cases control the illness. I have been diagnosed as suffering from this illness 24 years ago. Since then the only inconvenience I experienced was that I had to take one tablet a day. Am I sick? Technically yes, practically no.

[13] My elder brother is suffering from (incurable) Parkinson disease, but various medicines and a brain implant have considerably slowed down the progress of the illness and alleviated many (but not all) symptoms.

as healing) and observable facts. I do not think that always scientific or laboratory proof is required, observed healing may well be sufficient.[14]

In this book I will apply this terminology to HIV/Aids: Healing means that the illness is eliminated. Scientific medicine argues that such a healing for HIV/Aids is not (yet) possible. Many faith healers claim that it is, and some traditional healers made or make the same claim, in one case at least the claim was even for level (1) healing that included immunity after healing.

I will measure both traditional and Christian healers against their own claim to provide healing on levels (2) and (1), both involving elimination of the infection. Medical ("Western") science claims that only levels (3) control of and (4) alleviation can be currently achieved through Antiretroviral Treatment (ART). Another "Western" medical intervention is the Voluntary Male Medical Circumcision Campaign (VMMCC), which does not promise healing but the prevention of infection, and prevention of infection, in a way, would be the best form of healing. I will call this the (0) level of healing.

At the outset I must make it clear that in this book I am not dealing with psychological healing (healing of soul and mind without the removal of the illness) and social healing (the restoration of broken relationships),[15] and also not with spiritual healing.[16] Neither is this a book on the value

---

[14] I may offer my own experience here: I had been suffering from light but recurrent headaches, often 3 or 4 times a week, in 1990. That was never treated, but when my treatment for high blood pressure ("BP") started, the recurrent headaches disappeared. I still have occasional headaches, but not of that recurrent type. It may be difficult to prove scientifically the connection between the BP medicine and its effects on my headaches, but I am quite willing to see that as real healing.

[15] It is claimed that this restoration of broken relationships is a strength of African Traditional Healing, and there is some evidence for it, but when a traditional healer or diviner identifies the witch (normally a relative), who has caused a specific death, the opposite is true. In the olden days harmony in the community was sometimes restored by killing the perpetrator through the *mwabvi* poison ordeal. These days the same is sometimes attempted by expelling the accused from the village (especially if the accused is a widow who controls some land (Bridget Manda, Women and Witchcraft Accusations: A Case of Zomba Urban, MA Module, Mzuzu University, 2011).

[16] Such healing may take place in the case of a dying person who accepts salvation in Jesus Christ. A real life example: A mother of four wrote a kind of diary during the last two weeks of her life. She had been infected by her

of traditional (herbal) healing in general[17] nor about Christian healing in general; it only deals with healing (or non-healing) of HIV and AIDS.

1.2 The areas treated in this book

As the heading indicates, this book is not a dispassionate description of what people do when confronted with HIV infection, but a passionate study of fake healing claims. I will start with those that have a traditional religious background, then move to those systems which claim a scientific (herbal) base, followed by faith healing, and finally I will deal with the Voluntary Male Medical Circumcision Campaign, which offers no healing but prevention.

I am passionate about the issue as people die from fake healing claims, and that at a time when practical healing on level (3) is widely available, if not to all at least to so many. I am a theologian, and I feel obliged to develop a theology of the victims.[18] As a theologian I appreciate the discussion of fundamental truths, but only if such truths help those who suffer and do not kill them or spread the HIV infection further.

For each system of healing I will show the fundamental truth and analyze how this translates into (non-)healing on levels (0), (1) and (2). Some of the evidence comes from my own observation, some from

---

husband and the third TB treatment could not help her any more, and ARVs were not yet available. In the diary she forgave her husband for infecting her. The husband received and preserved the diary. I am not sure if he was healed spiritually, but his wife was healed indeed.

[17] While I was in Southern Tanzania, two young children of Jennifer and Habakuk Hallai fell sick with polio. The mission hospital could not help them, they went to a traditional doctor in the lakeshore area (Lake Nyasa) for an extended treatment, and they returned with both boys healed. This healing was certified by the mission doctor and was obvious to anyone who knew the family, myself included.

[18] See my articles: "'We are all Infected or Affected' - The Moralities of Antiretroviral Treatment", *Journal of Humanities*, no. 18 (2004), pp 19-37"; "Access to ARVs and the Role of the Churches", in *Religion in Malawi*, no. 12, 2005, pp. 6-10; "The Moralities of Condom Use. Theological Considerations," *Religion in Malawi* 2006, pp. 32-37; "Compulsory HIV Testing. A Christian Imperative," *Religion in Malawi* no. 14, 2007, pp. 33-39. The latter two have been reprinted and revised in Klaus Fiedler, *Conflicted Power in Malawian Christianity. Essays Missionary and Evangelical from Malawi*, Mzuzu: Mzuni Press, 2015, pp. 22-49.

existing literature and much from research my students in the Department of Theology and Religious Studies at Mzuzu University have done.

In view of the sources I have used, it is clear that my book does not offer a complete coverage of the phenomena discussed and that the random sampling used in it does not always fulfill the theoretical requirements for a sample to represent the whole. I am aware of these limitations, and since no one has presented a comprehensive study, I offer my observations for further scrutiny. From what I and others have observed I conclude that the healing claims dealt with in this book are fake and destructive. I would be happy to find contrary evidence.

2. Traditional healing claims

2.1 Chisupe

Having lived in Zomba for less than three years, I observed the eruption of Chisupe (or Mchape, as people soon began to name the medicine that Chisupe never named himself). I was so impressed by the many lorries that passed by the road behind my Kachere house leading to Liwonde, and, being a railway fan, I was impressed that on two Saturdays the Malawian Railways sent a special train to take the people from Blantyre there.

2.1.1 My sources

My interpretation is based on three levels of information: (1) My own observations (2) Joe DeGabriele's interview with Chisupe in 1996,[19] and (3) Three interpretative articles.[20] Joe DeGabriele focuses on the person and the ideas of Chisupe and draws attention to his views that

---

[19] Published as Kachere Documents no. 163: Joe DeGabriele, *Chisupe, Old Peppers don't Bite*, Zomba: Kachere, 1996.

[20] Matthew Schoffeleers, "The AIDS Pandemic, the Prophet Billy Chisupe, and the Democratization Process in Malawi," *Journal of Religion in Africa*, vol 29:4, pp. 406-441; Peter Probst, "'Mchape' '95, or, the Sudden Fame of Billy Goodson Chisupe: Healing, Social Memory and the Enigma of the Public Sphere in Post-Banda Malawi," *Africa*, Vol. 69, no 1, (1999), pp. 108-137; Marissa Doran, "Reconstructing Mchape '95: AIDS, Billy Chisupe, and the Politics of Persuasion," *Journal of Eastern African Studies*, 1:3, pp 397-416, published online 10.10.2007.

traditional society of old was morally clean and that the way forward would be a return to that morality where one man has one wife and is faithful to her. Schoffeleers sees the Chisupe event as a societal quest for moral purification,[21] while Probst sees Chisupe mainly as a new expression of the recurrent idea of witch finding and witch cleansing. Marissa Doran picks up Joe DeGabriele's observation that Chisupe was very concerned about the cultural and moral decline and makes this the tool of her interpretation.[22]

2.1.2 The events

Billy Goodson Chisupe, born 1916 in Kwipulu Village, TA Chikowi, Zomba District, had a vivid dream on 22.8.1994, in which his maternal uncle and a faceless figure appeared to him, asking him to go to a specific tree, cut its bark and administer it to anyone (free of charge) as a medicine to cure the incurable illness of Aids. He was not to take it to any other place or pass the cure on to others. With a flour offering he asked the spirits to come to him to give further explanations, which they did, and after that Chisupe quietly began to administer the concoction.

He and his medicine became famous when the MBC Radio programme "Morning Basket" gave him prominence, with people coming to him by the thousands a day. Estimates of the numbers of people who drank the medicine vary between 400,000 and 1,000,000.[23] The rush seems to have peaked within a few months, as in September 1995 "he was

---

[21] I disagree with Matthew Schoffeleers that the fact that there was no healing does not really matter.

[22] Chisupe was a "political strategist who used the media and the vehicle of AIDS to articulate a pointed critique of colonialism and neocolonialism" (Marissa Doran, "Reconstructing Mchape '95: AIDS, Billy Chisupe, and the Politics of Persuasion," *Journal of Eastern African Studies*, 1:3, pp 397-416 [407]). My problem with this interpretation is the ideological overload.

[23] That would mean 5% of the then population of Malawi or more. Numbers of visitors came from other Southern African countries.

receiving far fewer clients."[24] Still, while Joe DeGabriele was interviewing him for two hours in 1996, two men came to drink the medicine.[25]

2.1.3 The claims

Chisupe's claims were very clear: The medicine (with no name) would both heal AIDS (healing level 2) and would provide immunity (healing level 1). He maintained this claim even in view of the fact that no healings had occurred after more than a year. While insisting on the provision of immunity, he also insisted on moral reform (no adultery after healing).[26] Though the spirits had made the medicine dependent on him, he was ready to have its ingredients tested in a laboratory, at least in the beginning. The spirits had also told him to require those who drank the medicine to go to the hospital to get tested to prove their healing.[27]

2.1.4 The source of healing

Chisupe was a Christian, a member of the (Baptist) Providence Industrial Mission,[28] and I see no reason to doubt his Christian faith. Still, the appearances of the spirits of his relatives in the two dreams are clearly patterned after Traditional religious concepts. Traditionally, healers often receive their healing knowledge and powers in a dream. He emphasized that he was a healer, not a doctor (*sing'anga*), as he was

---

[24] Peter Probst, "'Mchape' '95, or, the Sudden Fame of Billy Goodson Chisupe: Healing, Social Memory and the Enigma of the Public Sphere in Post-Banda Malawi," *Africa*, Vol. 69, no 1, (1999), pp. 108-137 [116].

[25] Chisupe continued to administer the medicine until his death in 2004, after which his son took over.

[26] Marissa Doran dismisses this demand as an outside addition to his own words (p. 404), but Joe DeGabriele's report proves this as genuine. Marissa Doran seems to assume that in a person there can be no major inconsistencies, an assumption which I do not share.

[27] Probably a few gave blood samples to government, but if they did, no results were ever released.

[28] The official name of the church is "African Baptist Assembly," a daughter of the (Black) National Baptist Convention, Inc in the USA, of which John Chilembwe was the first missionary. (For the history see Patrick Makondesa, *The Church History of Providence Industrial Mission 1900-1940*, Zomba: Kachere, 2006).

given only one medicine, and he was not charging for his services as others were doing.[29] Chisupe was clearly convinced that the healing was granted by God. He was not a herbalist, as the medicine was dependent on him (or his family) administering it. This spiritual quality differentiates it from the later medicines of Chambe and Garani MW1, for which the inventors (or discoverers?) made only scientific claims.

2.1.5 The success

From all Chisupe said it is clear that the medicine would not bring improvement (healing level 4), but full healing with full immunity (level 1). In the newspapers I read in those days there was no report of anyone claiming or testifying to have been healed. The strongest claim that came to my notice was that someone said that every time he drinks the medicine, he "feels much better."[30] In spite of no healings, Chisupe continued to believe in the effectiveness of the medicine, and he continued to administer it until he died.

Though Chisupe did not explicitly deny that his medicine was effective to heal (or improve) other illnesses, he never saw it as multi-purpose or cure-all medicine.[31]

2.1.6 The false truth

At the height of the Chisupe affair, one of my theology students handed in a brief paper with the claim that God can reveal the cure for AIDS to an African. He was very angry that the *Azungu*[32] refused to recognize that. He had no doubts that Chisupe had been given that revelation. While I have no doubts that God can reveal a cure for AIDS to an African as much as to a *Mzungu*, the problem is that there is no indication that God has done so. Chisupe also claimed divine revelation, through the ancestors, but the problem is that there was no healing.

---

[29] There were several such healers in Southern Malawi around the same time, who had few clients and made no major impression on society.

[30] The sprits had said that one cup is enough, but over time Chisupe allowed repeats, and he also sometimes varied the dosage between 1 and 3 cups (but never more). He also tolerated that patients would settle for a time at his place in *misasa* (temporary grass shelters). Having "misasa patients" brought him closer to the traditional *sing'anga*.

[31] This claim is being made for Garani MW1.

[32] Azungu are the white people. The term is descriptive, not negative.

At the time of Chisupe there were no ARVs yet, so his false claims may not have done much damage to those infected. The claim of providing immunity against HIV infections could, in theory, have led to increased promiscuity, but at that time I heard nothing about that, and even in the literature available to me, there is no evidence of change in sexual behaviour, just as much as there is no evidence that his demand that there should be no promiscuity after drinking the medicine has had any effects.

Chisupe's medicine, initially called "water of life" provided people with hope, but a hope that would soon be disappointed.

2.1.7 Interpretations

There are four scholars who wrote about Chisupe, and their interpretations differed widely, spanning from societal cleansing to the fight against neocolonialism. My problem with these interpretations, each of which captures an interesting aspect, is that in none of them healing plays a role, and healing was the reason why half a million people went to see him. So I see the movement how the people saw it, I see it as a healing movement, albeit a failed one. If that is accepted, there is room to see other aspects as well. Joe DeGabriele points out Chisupe's view of the decline of morality, a decline brought about by intruding foreigners and by intruding foreign concepts.[33] Marissa Daren then makes him a politician fighting colonialism and neo-colonialism. I see little room for the societal cleansing aspect as argued by Schoffeleers, but maybe there was some experience of *communitas* with everyone, big and small, getting down to the same level, just wanting and getting the cup.

When I observed the events, I felt that there were many similarities to the Mchape witchcraft eradication movement of the 1930s and similar eradication movements after that. Chisupe never saw himself in that way, and he refused to equate AIDS with witchcraft. Therefore I can not see Chisupe as a witchcraft eradicator, but I may still point out some relationships, and I am supported in seeing these by the fact that the people called the medicine *muchape* (though Chisupe never did that).[34]

---

[33] In spite of these anti-white declarations Joe DeGabriele felt only warmth and no hostility during the interview.

[34] Peter Probst also picks up that relationship, and this becomes the main point of his interpretation. Probst points out correctly that Joe Chakanza, my colleague at that time and a specialist in witchcraft eradication movements, did not see that connection.

My main point to relate the two movements is that they both fought (seriously and without success) against the greatest evil in society, which was witchcraft for Mchape and AIDS for Chisupe. Once this point is accepted, other differences become minor: The old Muchape travelled, Chisupe was forbidden to do so. This can be explained by the changing circumstances of transport and (radio) communication. And for this change the witchcraft eradicator Nchimi Chikanga could lend some support, as he also, once at a place, waited for patients to come, and they came in great numbers.[35] He also did not charge for his treatments.

2.2 Sing'anga

At the time of Chisupe there were other healers who claimed to heal AIDS. The newspapers reported of two practitioners in Southern Malawi who offered full healing against proper payment. They had few people coming to them. They never caught the public imagination, and news about them did not continue.[36]

A few years later I saw along the Lilongwe – Likuni road three signs of *asing'anga* that claimed to heal AIDS. A number of years later I passed by again but did not find the signs there.

Since years the regular newspapers carry adverts about herbal medicine. This made the Nation newspaper publish regularly a disclaimer:

> We wish to advise our valued readers and advertisers that according to the medical profession, HIV/AIDS has no known cure yet. As a result, all claims by any parties to the contrary do not have any endorsement by Nation Publications Limited.[37]

In recent issues I could not find any advert that directly claimed healing for HIV/AIDS.[38] Nevertheless recently there was a statement by the

---

[35] Boston Soko, *Nchimi Chikanga. The Battle against Witchcraft in Malawi*, Blantyre: CLAIM-Kachere, 2002, ²2003.

[36] I have no copies of the newspapers; the Chisupe literature mentions them but gives no details.

[37] *Nation on Sunday*, 7.7.2015.

[38] It is all about finding lost love, getting rich, manhood enlarger, getting pregnant within four weeks (guaranteed and payment afterwards), solving financial problems etc. The only hint to HIV/AIDS I found in the Sunday Times of 26.7.2015 where World Herbals offer not only to enlarge the manhood and boost the hips, but also "antivirus blood cleaner." Towards the end of 2015 there came regular adverts from Dr Mama Amina, who offered the usual

executive director Davie Kalomba that making such adverts is wrong, "they are mostly unfounded because the said concoctions have not been scientifically proven to validate their claimed curative values."[39]

3. Chambe: "Healing the Nations"

After the excitement over Chisupe's promise of healing had been disappointed, a Malawian from South Africa provided new hope,[40] when he arrived in Malawi with the claim that in South Africa he had developed a herbal drug to heal HIV/AIDS, which had had great success there.[41] He now wanted to bring the same healing to Malawi.

The motto displayed was "Healing the Nations."[42] The product to achieve this was a brown concoction for which no details were ever given. Different from Chisupe's this was not a "one cup is enough" treatment, but a medicine to be taken over a time. I am not aware that publicly a "regular" time was announced for healing to take place. This, of course, makes any measurement of success difficult.

The other difference to Chisupe was that Chambe was a medicine to be sold, so that it largely became an urban and educated people's phenomenon. Chambe's successes were claims, but no evidence was provided. Over the years that led to the decline in its customer base. Now Chambe

---

"Finding lost lovers" (24 hrs), Manhood enlargement (big, strong and hardness), high blood pressure and diabetes etc, to which she added a rider: "NB: HIV/AIDS on symptoms" which I understand to be a disclaimer that she can not heal HIV/AIDS (*The Nation*, 12.11.2015).

[39] "Discovery of HIV and AIDS was a science, so there has to be an evidence scientifically to prove that whatever concoction someone has is able to cure AIDS. If one is sure that their medicine is able to cure HIV and AIDS, why not subject the same to the scientific test?" (Davie Kalomba's words as reported in *The Nation*, 5.8.2015, on the title page.)

[40] Here I base most of what I write on my memory and observation. I have not found any scholarly study of the phenomenon yet. So the main source are the newspapers, which unfortunately I did not keep.

[41] From all the reports about him it becomes in no way clear what happened to his healing business in South Africa.

[42] I remember well the big banner displayed over several years at the main road out of Lilongwe to the south, where the Chambe medicine was sold. (The banner is no longer there.)

seems to have petered out and I don't know of any banner still flying "Chambe – Healing the Nations."

An interesting twist in the story was the founder's conversion, to be born again. At conversion he decided to pass on the business to someone else. He seems to have not been comfortable with his business in his new status, though he explicitly stated that the medicine was indeed true.

As with Chisupe there was controversy over scientific testing, and as with Chisupe before and Garani MW1 afterwards there was no laboratory testing of the drug, and just as with Chisupe, no one did stand up with the claim: "I have been healed, do test me now."[43]

Popular enthusiasm there was, and quite some business. As is often the case when promises are not kept, a secondary message is offered to explain the failure. So what was a product for healing HIV/AIDS was now offered as an immune booster, not offering any longer healing on levels 1 and 2, but alleviation on level 4. The same happened with Chisupe's medicine. No one testified to healing, but there were several claims that its repeated use was helpful. The next step from here is seen in Garani MW1, which, originally designed against HIV/AIDS, developed into a "cure all" medicine.[44]

What did Chambe achieve? Definitely the nations were not healed. Neither were individuals. The damage was limited since ARVs were not yet accessible at that time, though the emotional damage of disappointed hopes should not be seen as negligible.

The Chambe medicine made no religious claims. Chisupe had administered a herbal drink and was willing to have it tested in a laboratory at one point, but he insisted that this (effective) herbal medicine only worked through him, thus making a claim of having received a divine revelation. For the Chambe medicine no such claims were made. For Chambe the healing agent was purely herbal, but it has in common the fact that, like with other mixed origin health products, none was healed and no conclusive evidence was provided or found of the immune boosting qualities.

---

[43] There are many arguments for demanding or refusing scientific (laboratory) testing. But before that a "field test" would provide initial evidence (negative for all these).

[44] That would be the first of its kind in world history. – For Garani MW1 the claim is not that it can cure one illness, but many.

4. A comparison: mixed agency healing claims outside Malawi

4.1. A herbal medicine from Tanzania and Congo

In the 1990s in Tanzania a herbal medicine was developed (or discovered?) to treat HIV/AIDS. It was much present in the Tanzanian press. A co-operation was established with Kinshasa University. Repeatedly initial successes were proclaimed and then the information stopped. No reason was given. I guess that the scientific tests did not find the healing properties.[45]

4.2. Rev Ambilikile Mwasapile, Tanzania

In 2011 Ambilikile Mwasapile, born c. 1935, a retired Lutheran Pastor in Northern Tanzania (Samunge Village, in Loliondo, near Ngorongoro) announced his mixed source healing capacities. God had shown him, like Chisupe, a tree (*mugariga*), that would heal "various chronic diseases" including cancer, high blood pressure, diabetes, and of course HIV/AIDS. Like Chisupe he offered a herbal drink that, with prayer (his prayers), would heal HIV/AIDS and several other diseases. Again, the healing was localized to his home, with tremendous traffic problems as he lived in a somewhat remote area. His medicine was sold, unlike Chisupe's, but since it was sold at 0.03 $, it was virtually free, like Chisupe's. The number of drug takers was in the hundred thousands. And like with Chisupe and Chambe, "foreigners came, even from Botswana," and even people in high positions came. His church did not disown him (neither did it endorse him), but the medical authorities did.[46] And like with Chisupe and Chambe, in all the fuss no healings were recorded.[47] And as with Chisupe, the place became much quieter after some time.

---

[45] The information for this paragraph is based on my memory of the reports in *Tanzania Information*, published by Mission Eine Welt, Neuendettelsau, which gives monthly reports about the Tanzanian Press. I have not kept these reports.

[46] The information comes from Marilyn Wouters, "Faith Healing in Simunge, Sonja Territory," on the web, May 2011, from Wikipedia ("Ambilikile Mwasapile").

[47] My information is limited to what I find on the web and my reading of various entries over time in the *Tanzania Nachrichtendienst.*" There were many reports about the crowds surging in on the village, but never a specific healing claim has come to my notice.

4.3 Prophet Stephen Kwagala, Uganda

Currently mixed sources healing is propagated on radio by a pastor who calls himself "Prophet Stephen Kwagala." His mixed sources are: faith and holy oils, and after the healing he refers the patients, so he claims, to a professional doctor "to seek further expertise proof."[48] He discovered his healing powers when he was preaching, and a woman suffering from HIV/AIDS was listening intently. "At once, she knew I can cure her ... I first prayed for her. I then washed her right leg with the anointed oil."[49].

5. Recent variants of multiple cure herbal drugs in Malawi

5.1 Teras!! The Wonderful Drug

While walking to the Greenshop in Mzuzu, I passed a shop advertising the drug Teras that cures "Cancer, Diabetes, Stroke, Heart and Kidney Failure, B.P., Fertility Problems etc."[50] I have not seen any advertising to it and I have not heard of any cancer patient testifying that she had been healed by the drug. In the shop advert there was no offer of healing HIV/AIDS, but if a drug can heal cancer (and several other potentially terminal illnesses), maybe it can even heal HIV/AIDS?

Later I learnt from the internet that this drug is composed of "spices, vegetables and fruits which are obtained locally." The owner is Shalice

---

[48] www.investigator.co.ug/crime/item/14983-ugandan-born-again - I see that this is a partisan source, but if many people had been healed, the news would have splashed about.

[49] Here again the website is my only source, which I can not crosscheck. But it follows a general trend. The website lists other forms of fake healing: It refers to an illiterate woman known as Nanyonga, in Ssembule in South Western Uganda, who "made a killing, selling bare soil, which she claimed could cure HIV." After Nanyonga came Mariandina promoted by an "internationally reputed medical consultant Dr Charles Ssali," who was publicly disowned by the Royal College of Surgeons of Edinburgh (http://www.independent.co.uk/news/doctor-earns-rebuke-for-aids-remedy-1167079.html).

[50] There are phone numbers displayed for Blantyre, Lilongwe and Mzuzu (My visit there 1.8.2015).

Amos, and a bottle costs MK 10,000. Teras can not heal HIV (as "that is a virus"), but it can heal AIDS, "as that is an illness."[51] For severe conditions six months of treatment are required, for lighter afflictions four months are enough. Teras is indeed a multipurpose dug, and it has been recognized by the Malawian Diabetes Society, "because of its proven effects."[52] Then the rider is added: "Do not stop regular prescribed treatment." So a healing drug (Level 1, which can heal AIDS!) has now been recognized as a food supplement!

5.2 Gloria Jeremiah's Herbal Hospital

I observed this offer of a double cure earlier last year. My wife and I had been travelling and when we spent a few days in the Zomba area, when returning from Blantyre, she received a phone call to help a lady from her home area with transport money to travel back to Mzuzu, and very urgently so, as she was very sick and the night bus would leave in a few hours. My wife preferred to see her first, and immediately hired a taxi to take her back to Mzuzu, as she probably would not have survived the bus journey.[53]

Here is the story behind this: While in Mzuzu she had been diagnosed with cancer, and all medical treatment had failed. Seeing that there was no help from Western medicine, her husband and the family sent her, with the required female guardian, to Gloria Jeremiah's Herbal Hospital, not far from Zomba. There she was admitted and treated with herbal medicine, with her health continuously deteriorating. When death was close, she was "transferred" to Zomba Central Hospital.[54] After a few days doctors decided that she should be taken home.[55] One may

---

[51] "HIV is a virus and our drug does not cure that, but it cures Aids which is a group of health problems that make up a disease due to weak immune system. Our drug is made of spices, vegetables and fruits which are obtained locally."

[52] www.nyasatimes.com/diabetes-association-of-malawi-endorses-teras-herbal-drug-with-stearn warning.

[53] She died 24 hrs after arrival in Mzuzu.

[54] The reason seemed to me to avoid her dying at the Herbal Hospital.

[55] Here the reason seemed to me that they felt it would be better for her and for her relatives that she should die at home (technically she was referred to Mzuzu Central Hospital "to continue the treatment").

understand that her husband and family, after all "Western" medical help had failed, tried what offered the only hope and invested the money and care into finding that way. But one may not understand that an herbal hospital treats her for three months without any hope of healing and sends her away after a total failure to die elsewhere. This appears to be gross abuse. I have not learnt which herbal treatment this lady received, probably not Garani MW1, but such practices throw a very bad light on the healing claims of Mrs Jeremiah's Herbal Hospital.[56]

5.3 The Hospital of Creation (Chipatala cha Chilengedwe)[57]

This is a book that offers teaching for healing over 120 illnesses. It was written from a religious background,[58] but the treatments offered have no religious preconditions in themselves.

---

[56] "The fact that supposedly reputable newspapers in Malawi have chosen to give the claims credence with sycophantic and sensationalist reporting is particularly appalling. It is the kind of reporting that causes real damage and costs lives. It should be condemned." – This is the concluding judgment in: Sintha Chiumia/Julian Rademeyer, "Claim that Malawi 'wonder herb' cures HIV is untrue and irresponsible"(https://africacheck.org/reports/claim-that-...., published 9.6.2013, accessed 8.10.2016).

[57] Langford L. Dzanja, *Chipatala cha Chilengedwe. Machiritso Kupyolera Mu Chilengedwe. 1*, np., Advent Publications, nd [2014]. The name "Advent Publications" does not involve any endorsement by the Seventh-day Adventist Church. But the book shows that there is *some* affinity to the Adventist health message. To study the SDA health message see: Frank Chirwa, Theology of Health in the Seventh-day Adventist Church: A Quest for Abundant Life in Jesus, Mzuni Documents no. 112, 2010. The SDA hospitals show no aversion at all against ARVs.

[58] This is expressed in a quotation on the cover from Rev 22:2 "And the leaves from the tree are for the healing of the nations" ("Ndipo masamba a mtengo ndiwo akuchiritsa nawo amitundu") and also in the problematic note on AIDS: "Lingalirani pomwe simunachite bwino, pamene panapangitsa kuti mutenge nthendayi.—Consider where you did not behave well, so that you contracted the disease." (This is a very harsh advice for wives who were infected by their husbands in their marriage bed.) I also have problems with the final biblical quote from 2 Kings 5:10 where Eliza tells the Syrian general to submerge himself seven times in the river Jordan to receive a miraculous divine cure for leprosy (in those days leprosy was probably as stigmatized as HIV/AIDS is today.)

The text does not *explicitly* claim that the herbal and food prescriptions can *heal* AIDS, but "Aloe Vera will help to stop the multiplication of the virus, and Moringa, taken 3x daily, will increase the immune power, and garlic kills the virus," and while for stomach cancer the first thing to be done is to see a doctor, for HIV there is no hint to that or that ARVs can prolong life. (From this I must assume that ARVs are not needed in the "Hospital of Creation.")

In the book there are 12 pages for the treatment of various forms of cancer. For stomach cancer, of which my mother died, a patient is requested to see a hospital doctor, to avoid inappropriate food, and to eat appropriate food like lentils, broccoli, Brussels sprouts, and not to forget flaxseed and garlic and to drink pineapple juice.[59]

5.4 Wizika

A new herbal drug has just been discovered, called Wizika, produced by a "Dr Kaunda" and "applied successfully" at his Herbal Clinic at Chintheche.[60] It is a multi-purpose drug able to cure HIV but not AIDS, as "AIDS is too advanced."[61] Different from Chisupe and others, one cup is not enough, and to be cured from HIV (though not from AIDS), three months or more are needed. Like with Chisupe and Chambe, patients come "even from South Africa and Botswana." The drug is not free, but priced at MK 1,500 it is not expensive compared to Chambe and Garani MW1. As much as Chisupe claimed to have healed a white lady, "Dr" Writing Zigowe Kaunda cured an American, Dr Jeffy Metzger, of diabetes, five years ago.[62] And Metzger took Wizika with him to America for laboratory tests, "which are progressing" and the "medicine is curing people." So the drug will be "on the world market and will enjoy massive

---

[59] Langford L. Dzanja, *Chipatala cha Chilengedwe. Machiritso Kupyolera Mu Chilengedwe,* no place: Advent Publications, nd [2014], p. 96.

[60] Tendayi Chvyunguma, "Exit Mchape and Chambe, enters Wizika. Malawian Herbalist Claims" (malawi24.com/2015/05/23/exit-mchape-and-chambe-enters-wizika, accessed 20.7.2015, 7.10.2016 and 28.11.2016).

[61] Opposite to this, Teras, the wonderful drug, can heal AIDS but not HIV.

[62] Jeff Metzger, ND, works in private naturopathic medical practice ("Jeff Metzger, ND", www.seattledigestivehealth.com) and also teaches at Bastyr University, a university for alternative (naturopathic) medicine (bastyr.edu). — Neither website mentions anything about Wizika nor about treating or healing HIV/AIDS. Both websites accessed 28.11.2016.

publicity."[63] Like Gloria Jeremiah he complains that the Ministry of Health, after receiving the drug, refuses to test it.[64]

5.5 The false truth about herbs healing HIV/AIDS

My student in Zomba in the days of Chisupe commented (angrily), why the *azungu* were not willing to believe that God had revealed the cure for AIDS to an African. I do believe that God can do that, but whatever was revealed to Chisupe in his dreams, it was no cure for HIV/AIDS. How beautiful would it have been!

The same applies to herbs, unfortified by faith. I know that there is healing in many herbs, plants and roots. And I would be so happy if, like with quinine for malaria, a powerful herb could be found. The problem is that it has not been found, for which numerous healings would be the proof,[65] not emphatic claims. I would be so happy if the herb would be found.

6. Faith Healing HIV/AIDS

6.1 The false truth

I do believe that God heals, not only through the dedicated work of doctors and nurses, or through the various medicines, be they herbal, mineral or chemical, but sometimes also in miraculous ways as an answer to prayer and faith. Such healings are attested to in the Old and New Testament,[66] through various periods of Church History and even now they are there.[67]

---

[63] Currently there are about 10 Million people on ARVs in Africa, with massive positive results, so Wizika will have a lot of competition.

[64] The information I have on Wizika is from only one website, so I can not guarantee its reliability. But the information fits a common pattern and is probably correct.

[65] If there were such numerous healings, lab tests would follow easily.

[66] There is one rationalistic strand in Presbyterian theology (especially in America), which argues that the miraculous gifts like speaking in tongues and prophecy, miracles and healing, had been designed by God to verify the Christian revelation and were withdrawn by God after that revelation was written down in the biblical canon. Among such cessationist theologians there is

In my study of the Faith Missions I found not only the Holiness Movement, but as a branch of it also a Healing Movement and the literature attests to many healings over the years that could hardly have been explained otherwise.[68] These healings often took place in Healing Homes which those seeking healing attended for shorter or longer periods,[69] like Andrew Murray, the spiritual father of the early Nkhoma Mission.[70] Important is to observe that these Healing Homes put themselves to the test. Healing was not pronounced (and the patients then sent home) but experienced (and observed, failures included.)[71]

---

controversy about the gift of healing, as some are willing to concede that it may not have been completely withdrawn.

[67] An acquaintance of mine in Germany suffered from multiple sclerosis (MS), a slowly progressing incurable disease. She had been showing already visible symptoms. She was prayed for and healed, and all signs of MS left her never to return. She later worked as a nurse in an MS ward. The patients asked her why she could understand them so well. She never told them that she had been healed, as she had not received the gift of healing, so she did not want to put an additional burden on the patients. Her doctor did not believe in prayer, so he declared that her case was one of "spontaneous healing." There is no need to argue as he accepted that she was indeed healed.

[68] For my treatment of that Healing Movement see: Klaus Fiedler, *Ganz auf Vertrauen. Geschichte und Kirchenverständnis der Glaubensmissionen*, Gießen/Basel, Brunnen Verlag, 1992, pp. 78f, 85, 221, 231. Out of print, but available on http://tinyurl.com/fiedler for free download.

[69] In these healing homes there were many who were healed, but there were also some who finally left without being healed.

[70] As the pastor of Wellington DRC congregation he had lost, over many months, his ability to speak louder than with a whisper. Then he went to London, checked into Mrs Baxter's healing home, which he left after some time, being completely healed. For all the remaining years of his life, his voice never left him again and he could preach to the crowds as before the affliction (Andrew Murray, *Divine Healing. A Serious of Addresses and Personal Testimony,* London: Victory Press, 1900). For his life see: Leona Choy, *Andrew Murray. Apostle of Abiding Love*, Ft Washington: CLC, 1978; J. du Plessis, *The Life of Andrew Murray of South Africa,* London/Edinburgh/New York 1919. The web offers much information. A starting point would be: www.dacb.org/stories/southafrica/murray_jr.html.

[71] The biblical testimony contradicts the healing practice of the "prophets" mentioned, because all miracles in the bible were instant healings, publicly

A major centre of healing was Zion, Illinois, a newly founded city by Alexander Dowie, which by definition could have neither a doctor nor a pharmacy, and people were healed.[72] For Malawian Zionists, Zion Illinois is important as all the 30 Zionist denominations in Malawi trace their origins (through South Africa) to Zion, Illinois.[73]

I am convinced that God can and does heal people. I am also convinced that God can heal HIV/AIDS. But from all I know this is rare. Bishop Matoga of the Faith of God Church and a practicing healer, told me ten years ago that he knew of five cases of HIV/AIDS healing through faith.[74] Isabel Phiri also described a case of HIV/AIDS healing through prayer. And I think there may be some more. So the truth is confirmed that God can heal even HIV/AIDS. What makes the truth false is Its application. HIV patients are taken to Christian healers, they are prayed for, pronounced healed and dismissed, with the admonition (probably better: command) not to go to a hospital nor to take any ARVs, and a few months down the line they die (of the very same illness they had earlier been healed from). This turns the truth into a lie.

6.2 Some observations

A few of us were standing at the roadside in Chibavi, the next suburb to Chibanja, where we live in Mzuzu. I don't know how she came to talk to us and why she wanted to tell her story. She had been on ARVs, then she was prayed for, her status deteriorated ever after, until, in the nick of time, she saw the light and returned to her ARVs, which saved her life. But she had no good word for a healer whom she considered fake.

---

observed. And when Jesus pronounced the servant of the centurion healed, the centurion could go home and check, and he found him well (Lk 7:10). Neither Jesus nor the apostles ever said "You are healed now, but to keep your healing you must do this or that (and do not show yourself to the priests to be checked).

[72] When I visited Zion, Illinois, I asked my host how his family had come to Zion. He told me that his grandparents had a sick daughter and they asked Alexander Dowie to come and pray for her. Dowie did not do that, but arranged that at an exact time the parents and himself should pray for the girl. She was promptly healed, so her parents moved to Zion in gratitude.

[73] For a deep study of all the Zionist Churches in Malawi see Ulf Strohbehn, *The Zionist Churches in Malawi - History -Theology – Anthropology*, Mzuzu: Mzuni Press, 2016.

[74] He emphasized that no one prayed for may abandon the ARVs.

Around the same time there was a funeral in our vicinity, again in Chibavi. The lady had been prayed for, deteriorated regularly, was advised not to take ARVs again, just to have faith, and then she died. And the pastor who had "healed" her presided over her funeral.

While I taught in class about ARVs and HIV/AIDS, a student told me that an elder female relative of his had been prayed for and refuses to take medicine, but with her health deteriorating. I asked him to tell his aunt that she is playing with her life and that she will die soon unless she takes the ARVs again. The next semester he saw me again and told me that his aunt has started to take ARVs again, and "now she is much better."

One student asked me to be allowed to do research on the issue of faith healing and herbal healing: "I was motivated to conduct this research due to the death of my aunt who in 2005 tested HIV positive and was committed to ARV treatment immediately. She claimed to have been healed through prayer and abandoned ARV treatment on 4th December 2013, with effects of drug defaulting."[75]

6.3 Nahori Malisa's research

Nahori Malisa tried to verify the healing claims of both traditional and Christian healers of HIV/AIDS in the Charismatic context. He found a pastor who welcomed him to talk about HIV/AIDS healing, but when he was asked for any proof of healing, these words ended the interview:

> The problem with you students is that you don't believe in faith healing, therefore, I cannot produce the evidence you are looking for. Thank you.[76]

Nahori Malisa found and interviewed a number of women who claimed to have been healed of HIV/AIDS. All refused to have their healing tested. One answer was typical: "We can not go because doing so is demeaning our faith in God."[77]

All the women who claimed to have been healed refused to be tested. F1 had this to say:

---

[75] Nahori Malisa, Analyzing Critical HIV and AIDS Results in Malawi. A Case Study of an Interface between Christian Faith/Traditional Healing Claims and Scientific Treatment, BA, Mzuzu University.

[76] Interview with a Pentecostal Church pastor in Nkhotakota, [Nahori Malisa].

[77] Int F2 and F3 [Nahori Malisa].

> I cannot go to the hospital because I know my God has healed me. Can't you see that I am strong? If you insist that I go with you to the hospital for evidence, leave me alone and go! You cannot see this because you don't believe. I don't care about going to the hospital because I don't believe in it anymore.[78]

6.3.1 Healed to death

Nahori Malisa's sample is small, still, he found *claims* of healing but no one was willing to be tested, and he points out that the time to state healing without a laboratory test was simply too short. He found no evidence of healing, but solid evidence of two cases of "healing to death." A mother said about her daughter:

> I asked what made her stop taking ARVs; she said I received healing at Soul Winners Church in town. The Doctors could not save my daughter; it was too late because she cut off treatment in October 2012 leading to her death in January 2014.[79]

The next testimony is related:

> Jessie was my niece. I brought her up from her primary school days since her biological mother had died. We were together as a family enjoying our relationship until 2009 when she joined a certain church in town. She became too devoted to religious life and this was the period when her health was deteriorating. She accused me of practicing Satanism and attributed her ill health to this power. I was disappointed realizing the love I had on her as my own child and we stayed without talking to each other for four months. However, the mist was cleared when her situation worsened in 2010, she was very sick that I took her to Kamuzu Central Hospital where we were told that she was HIV positive and must immediately start ARVs. I was able to forgive her of what she accused me of having involvement in since I understood her desperation. She continued switching churches, a tendency I treated as normal to someone seeking forgiveness. She regained strength from the time she started taking ARVS until October 2012 when she began losing weight. She was hospitalized in April 2013 when it was discovered that she had not been taking ARVs, which led to liver problems, and the Doctors could not do anything to sustain her because it was too late a development

---

[78] Int F1 [Nahori Malisa].

[79] Int F11 [Nahori Malisa].

which led to her death. Before dying she said she was prayed for and was applied anointed oil on her fore head at Soul Winners in town.[80]

These stories about "healing to death" are not isolated, as I have heard a good (really: bad) number of them.

6.3.2 A newspaper report

On 2.2.2016 *The Nation* reported that in Bandawe five people died "after being advised by a pastor to abandon the life-prolonging treatment in Nkhata-Bay." T/A Malanda reported under tears that he lost his nephew "following the pastor's directive on the grounds that he was completely healed after a deliverance session administered to him."[81]

6.3.3 An assessment

I have no big statistical evidence, and I do not know of anyone who has such. But the evidence that is there is devastating:

> (1) There are healers (these days often called prophets) who claim to have or to mediate God's power of healing HIV/Aids.
>
> (2) They take no responsibility for their "healing."[82]
>
> (3) They take their own claims as the proof for their healings' effectiveness and do not allow testing.
>
> (4) People die of their "healing."
>
> (5) The name of Christ is damaged by those who claim to serve him.
>
> (6) A prophet, according to the Bible, is proven true or false by one simple fact: If his or her words do not come true, they are false prophets (Deuteronomy 18:21-22).[83]

---

[80] Interview Mrs Nkhoma [Nahori Malisa].

[81] T/A Malanda mentioned the name of the pastor, but it was not reported in the newspaper. I have no way to independently verify the events, but the details make the account credible.

[82] This was different with the healers in the Holiness Movement's Healing Houses, who stayed with their patients until they were proven as healed (and even if not).

(7) Often the divine healing is pronounced, but tied to conditions (Don't take ARVs, you must have faith, occasionally even tithing is such a requirement "to keep the healing" etc).[84]

(8) A recent development seems to be that, in some cases, the "cure" can be effected (only) by healing substances like Holy Water or Holy Anointments.[85]

(9) One may understand people's hopes for healing, but the self-destructive behaviour is difficult to explain, giving up proven treatment (level 3) for mere hope or mere promises.[86]

These deadly (or at least: dangerous) healing practices are frequent in certain sections of the Charismatic Movement in Malawi, but they are not shared by its majority. Living Waters, the biggest Charismatic church in Malawi, does emphasize prayer, but emphasizes that the taking of ARVs must not be stopped.[87] The same applies to Word Alive Ministry

---

[83] "You may say to yourselves, 'How can we know when a message has not been spoken by the LORD? If what a prophet proclaims in the name of the LORD does not take place or come true, that is a message the LORD has not spoken. That prophet has spoken presumptuously. Do not be afraid of him." [NIV]

[84] Occasionally the healing is tied to financial commitments like regular tithing (in an extreme case even to tithing to the ministry that has 'healed' the patient), and if tithing stops the illness comes back.

[85] Such holy substances are required for HIV healing in the case of Prophet Stephen Kwagala in Uganda (www.investigator.co.ug/crime/item14983). Recently a case from Mzuzu was reported in the newspaper, for an unspecified ailment, where the sufferer was required to buy MK 3000 healing oil and pay MK 21000 for holy anointing. Since the family was short of MK 3000 the healing could not take place. I do not generalize such stories. A very recent incident is the Prophet Shepherd Bushiri, originally from Northern Malawi, but now based in South Africa. He came with his "Shepherd Bushiri Aircraft" for a three day campaign to Mzuzu and was selling anointed water for MK 5000 and anointed oils for MK 10,000 (*Nation*, 26.9.2015).

[86] Nahori Malisa asked for the reasons, and these were stated by his respondents: (1) To avoid the social stigma of being infected (2) To avoid having to take the ARVs for life, considered to be inconvenient. (3) Fear of divorce (4) The wish not to prolong life a *little* (as ARVs promise "by maybe ten years"), but well beyond that. (5) To avoid "body disfigurement" (Nahori Malisa, p. 11).

[87] Personal Communication, Khetwayo Banda, Blantyre, Living Waters pastor, 2015.

International, the oldest Charismatic denomination,[88] and Bishop Matoga (Faith of God Church), who told me about five cases of HIV/AIDS healing through prayer, at the same time told me that no one, after being prayed for, must stop taking ARVs.

In spite of a strong amount of wisdom on this issue in the more established part of the Charismatic Movement, the Prophets flourish, and I have the impression that their number is growing. Here a clear and public dissociation from false prophets and healers (or whatever name they may take) is required by responsible leaders in the Charismatic Movement, but I have not come across any such public statements. After all the good name of Christ is at stake and the lives of many believers.[89]

6.4 Herbal HIV/AIDS medicine is less dangerous, but still...

Nahori Malisa equally investigated the healing claims of traditional healing. He met and interviewed Mrs Gloria Phiri, not in her hospital, but in Lilongwe. I feel it is worth quoting her at length because of the mixed messages the text contains:

> This is a herb that is treating people who have HIV and AIDS. The dosage is based on the experience of the person who was told about the medicine in a dream,[90] took it and got cured and the two of us are not the owners of this medicine and we are not herbalists. There is evidence that people who have taken our herb have gone to hospitals to get tested using tests like DNA/PCR test and antibody and the results have proven that they are negative. People come back with reports from the hospital in their health passports or lab forms and sometimes we photocopy the results at the clients' will. One bottle is taken within the period of 20 days and one month break is observed before taking another. One may repeat taking the herb in a month interval and for one to finish dosage, advisably; it should be a maximum of six bottles to be taken within ten months. We also advise our clients to

---

[88] Khetwayo Banda, Word Alive Ministries International (WAMI) and its Wholistic Mission, MA, Mzuzu University, 2012.

[89] Fortunately a good number of those who have deceived themselves or have been deceived, at some point see the light (and the truth) and return to ARVs, thus saving their lives. But why should they be deceived and suffer?

[90] For traditional medical practitioners it is not uncommon that they "receive" the healing medicine in a dream.

> continue taking medicine as prescribed by the hospital such as ARVs and Bactrim because Garani MW1 is not a replacement of ARVs. We advise our clients to abstain from sexual intercourse or use a condom during the period of treatment until they are proven negative by medical personnel at the hospital. Many people benefit from our treatment and yet the government allowed us to be selling to the public as a herb while waiting for research.[91]

Besides this interview Nahori Malisa was not given any evidence for any healing. But he found at least one woman who died because she relied on Garani MW1. Her husband reported:

> My wife and I tested HIV positive in 2009 ... My wife never came to terms with her status because she did nothing to contract HIV, I agree she was very faithful and it is me who infected her. One time, early 2013, she came joyfully that she had found medicine, which heals HIV and AIDS, meaning Garani MW1. I tried to reason with her that AIDS has no cure but she could not listen.[92] I suspect she stopped taking ARVS when she started taking the herb. This year in January [2014] she was very sick and when she could refuse medicine I thought it was due to her ill health. It came to my knowledge that she started defaulting on taking medicine long time ago, when I was told by the Doctor, and she died later in February 2014.[93]

This is the only "healing to death" report related to Garani MW1. This is still much more than "reliable healing reports," of which there is nothing but claims.

Interesting is Mrs Jeremiah's claim that her medicine heals HIV infection but scientific medicines like ARVs and Antibiotics must not be dropped. I

---

[91] Int. Mrs G. Jeremia (The Managing Director of Garani MW1 HIV and AIDS herb) who claims that this herb has power to heal AIDS because she has had experience regarding HIV issues for she is a professional in public health hence does not support any herb but this one alone [Nahori Malisa].

[92] According to Gloria Jeremiah those taking Garani should not stop taking ARVs, but—here as elsewhere—it is the listener who decides on the meaning of the message. See the same for the Voluntary Male Medical Circumcision Campaign with disastrous results. For a website intent on checking "alternative" healing claims see: https://africacheck.org/reports/a-roundup-of-fake-aids-cures-angels-zapper-garani-mw1-topvein-sf-2000/ (accessed 20.10.2016).

[93] Int. M1 (Mtsiliza HIV and AIDS support group) [Nahori Malisa].

also find it interesting that she has the records of people being healed, but instead of presenting them, she looks for government laboratory tests, of which she should be sure that they are not coming.[94]

Nahori Malisa summarizes his findings on herbal HIV/AIDS cures like this:

> Against the claims made by some traditional medicine practitioners that their medicine can heal HIV and AIDS, I found no evidence of any healing.

While he is very clear on this point, he found that possibly some of these herbal medicines may have nutritive value, as three women testified of "body figure replenishment" undoing side effects of ARV treatment. He proposes that these potential beneficial side effects should be scientifically investigated, not for healing HIV/AIDS, but for other benefits. The evidence he found would not be sufficient to claim healing on level (4) "alleviation."

6.5 The true truth about faith healing

Yes, God can heal HIV/AIDS, and I believe that he has done it. I am not refusing to recognize this truth statement, but I strongly object to change this truth into: "God will heal you of HIV/AIDS" as that puts the burden on the patient as she has to fulfill the conditions to achieve (or maybe sustain) the healing.[95]

Equally strongly I reject the instant declaration: "God has healed you of HIV/AIDS." I believe that God can heal HIV/Aids, but it happens infrequently, and definitely he did not give that power to this or that prophet for automatic application. The tragedy is that the healer does

---

[94] Albert Sharra, "Probing HIV Cure Herbs: Who is Losing?" *Weekend Nation*, 7.2.2015, pp. 20-21.—In the article the price tag for the test is given at MK 16,000,000.

[95] When I was pastor in Ratingen Baptist Church, we had as a church member a 15 year old girl in a wheel chair who had become disabled in a road accident at age seven. She was wheeled to a big healing convention some distance away, where the healer had devolved the healing prayers (due to big numbers) to others. The man who prayed for her said before the prayer: "It is quite possible that God will not heal you immediately, but he will surely do it if you continue to be thankful every day." As predicted, she was not healed, and who can expect a 15 year old girl in a wheelchair (or anyone of us walking straight on two feet!) to be thankful every day? Effectively she was blamed that she was destroying God's healing power. Similar gross abuse, where the victim is blamed for the failure of the healer, is frequent with some faith healers in Malawi.

not wait for the healing to be proven, and the healed person is not allowed to check for herself. The prophets use the Bible to claim that God has healed the person, but they ignore the fact that in the Bible patients were not "pronounced" healed but were *really* and *visibly* healed.[96]

This means that all those prophets (even if they have other titles) who pray for HIV/AIDS and require that ARVs be dropped, have no divine mandate and are false prophets as their pronouncements (predictions) do not come true. Even if they could produce a few patients who have indeed been healed (after sufficient time has elapsed and after they have been properly tested),[97] they are still false prophets, *who kill people in God's name*. They did not predict that *occasionally* someone might get healed, but that the individual just prayed for was (or would be) healed. A prophet is not proven true by occasionally getting a prediction right, but *all he predicts* must be right if he or she is a true prophet.[98]

6.6 What about ARVs?

I see it as tragic that in the name of God (whose name must not be abused) or in the name of the ancestors or in the name of (herbal) science people infected with HIV are made to suffer (or/and are making themselves to suffer) and sometimes even die, all that at a time when there is healing (albeit on level 3) available to anyone asking for it. Here again false "truths" come in: "ARVs only prolong life", "ARVs do not help everyone," etc. While these are truth, there is the equally scientific truth that millions of people have received healing on level 3 through them and that there are so many people in every location who, through being still alive, testify to the power of ARVs to offer healing that is real and saving lives. Yes, the virus is still in the body, but that is much more healing than being dead, be it through faith healing or herbal healing.

---

[96] Jesus even sent someone he had healed from leprosy (a term which in those days covered many skin diseases) to the priests to be declared healed ["clean"] (Luke 17:11-19). Neither Jesus nor Paul ever said "you must be thankful every day," "do not go to another doctor" or "buy some holy olive oil."

[97] I have not come across any such evidence yet and would be happy to find it.

[98] Here again Dt. 18:22 applies ("If what a prophet proclaims in the name of the LORD does not take place or come true, that is a message the Lord has not spoken. That prophet has spoken presumptuously.")

6.6.1 The sin of pride

Theologians say that the original sin of mankind is pride (hybris), wanting to be like God. As theologians we need to be thankful that God has given a level (3) remedy for HIV/AIDS that has dramatically changed the course of the pandemic. In Africa alone over 10,000,000 people are taking these drugs,[99] and while there is no 100% success, the death rates have gone down dramatically, extending the life span of millions.[100] This is proven healing, no lab tests are required, because many thousands of people in Malawi alone, who would be dead by now, are still alive and the majority of them with a quality of health that makes the illness undetectable for the outsider and who are able to work, enjoy life, bring up their children[101] and maybe even have another child or two.[102]

The opposite of the sin of pride (hybris) is humility, where man accepts his or her position as given by God, not trying to be like God and improve on his doings. Humility accepts gratefully what God has given, applies it to the benefit of all, and prays that God may give more.

6.6.2 The witchcraft connection

All over Malawi (and beyond) it is frequent to identify an (often unexplainable) illness as caused by witchcraft, originating mostly from within the extended family,[103] but also sometimes from neighbours or

---

[99] Out of above 15,000,000 worldwide (BBC News, July 2015).

[100] It is not yet known how many years the drug can extend a patient's life, as the drug is less than 20 years old, and people who took it right in the early years are still alive.

[101] Here the frequent biblical injunction to look after the widows and orphans comes into play. It is good to do right that, but the best way to fulfill this biblical command is to avoid that children become orphans and that their mothers die. Therefore not to take ARVs when they are (easily) available and rely on something of proven ineffectiveness (even if an occasional healing could be proven) is gross disobedience to God's command.

[102] For most people on ARVs the viral load is invisible. That does not mean that they are no longer infectious, but that the infectiousness is greatly reduced. Together with the regular prevention of mother to child infection the chance is very high (though not 100%) that an infected couple may give birth to HIV free children. I know a number of such children who are growing up healthily.

[103] I asked my 2014 Guidance and Counselling class to write down observations about an HIV/AIDS case within their observation or in which they took an

fellow employees. At this point theologians and scientists should equally be concerned. While the scientists aim should be to point out to the real causes of HIV, the theologians should be keenly concerned to protect the victims of witchcraft accusations. This story from one of the students tells it:

> My neighbour one day got very sick to the point that we people around her were very afraid that she was going to die. The entire family was suspecting her aunt to be bewitching her, but elder people around that area advised her to go to hospital and get diagnosed and see the way forward. After some discussion they agreed to go to the hospital. She was found positive and the CD4 count was very low, immediately they advised her to start taking ARVs and now she is healthy and the entire family refutes the claim that the aunt is a witch.

Is it not an act of honouring God helping someone through God given medicine and to free another one from (in some cases life-threatening) accusations? I suspect that some of the failing prophets fuel witchcraft suspicions and accusations by their teachings and in turn become failing (neo) traditional healers and equally useless deliverers as so many traditional doctors have become.

The students reported about 15 cases of healing (level 3) through ARVs, some for 10 years already, and 5 cases of non-healing through traditional healers and one case each of failed healing by prayer and by herbal medicine.[104]

7. The Voluntary Male Medical Circumcision Campaign

The Voluntary Male Medical Circumcision Campaign (VMMCC) does not claim to heal HIV/AIDS but to help in preventing the infection. Since prevention of an illness is better than any healing, I include VMMCC into this study, assigning it the healing level 0, a level that is better than cure and immunity on healing level 1. What applies to the other levels applies

---

initiative to help. 13 of the cases involved witchcraft, in 21 no witchcraft was mentioned (2 students did not report a case). This is not a scholarly test, but it shows how related HIV/AIDS and witchcraft are.

[104] Maybe the man who "had relied heavily on drugs from the pharmacy" may also have been taking herbal drugs.

here as well: Prevention, like healing, can not be proven by claims or theoretical arguments, but only by a decline in infections.[105]

7.1 The false truth of VMMCC

The false truth in this case is that VMMCC "reduces the chance of infection by up to 60%."[106] I checked with the current director of the Hospital for Tropical Diseases in Tübingen, and, of course she could not comment on "up to 60%," but she confirmed that indeed male circumcision reduces the chance of female to male HIV transmission.

As with other theoretical healing claims, this claim needs to be checked on the ground. Does the campaign which puts this claim on its banner as scientifically proven truth actually achieve a reduction in infections? The argument will be presented below, but before that my findings: While I appreciate the good intentions of the campaign, my observation is that VMMCC does not achieve a reduction in HIV infections but the opposite: **It promotes the spread of HIV/AIDS.**[107]

7.2 The international origin of the campaign in Malawi

VMMCC came to Malawi on recommendation of the World Health Organization and UNAIDS, who, at a meeting in Montreux, Switzerland (2007), accepting the findings of three randomized field trials conducted by circumcision proponents, officially promoted VMMCC "as an

---

[105] As big statistical evidence on a decline in the number of infections due to a specific intervention is difficult to produce, anecdotal evidence or small scale studies may help to verify or falsify claims of improved prevention.

[106] www.who.int/HIV/topics/male circumcision/en. I have not found out to which 100% these "up to 60%" refer. If it refers to the statistical average of unprotected sexual acts needed to get infected, the figure to contract an infection would rise by "up to 60%", but still leaving "40% or more" to get infected, while the protection rate of condoms is well over 90%. Alufandika also reported that nobody could tell him what 100% were, neither could he find it in the official reports available to him (Alufandika, p. 22 and p. 1). Maybe the figure includes the claim that every circumcised male must use condoms, and then the protection would rise from 98% to 99.2%.

[107] This chapter of my book is based on my own observations and the conclusions are mine, but most of the evidence comes again from my students' research, especially from Joseph Alufandika, The Voluntary Male Medical Circumcision (VMMCC) Campaign: Dissemination and Impact. A Case Study of T/A Mbenje in Nsanje, Southern Malawi, BA, Mzuzu University, 2013.

additional HIV prevention strategy" in the fight against AIDS."[108] VMMCC was adopted as an "additional prevention strategy."[109] If this idea is taken seriously, it would mean the usual ABC tools are kept (abstinence, faithfulness and condoms). Since condoms, if properly used, offer up to 98% protection, male circumcision would increase that to offer up to 99.2% protection.

In medical research randomized field trials are an accepted mode of testing medical theories. I am not a medical researcher, but my doubts about the validity of the field trials are supported by much adverse publicity. Alufandika refers to a number of such articles, including a statement by 40 senior health officials in South Africa that the randomized field trials there do not form a basis to advocate a large scale circumcision campaign.[110]

---

[108] Joseph Alufandika, The Voluntary Male Medical Circumcision (VMMC) Campaign: Dissemination and Impact. A Case Study of T/A Mbenje in Nsanje, Southern Malawi, BA, Mzuzu University, 2013.

[109] The current text on the WHO website reads: "There is compelling evidence that male circumcision reduces the risk of heterosexually acquired HIV infection in men by approximately 60%. Three randomized controlled trials have shown that male circumcision provided by well trained health professionals in properly equipped settings is safe. WHO/UNAIDS recommendations emphasize that male circumcision should be considered an efficacious intervention for HIV prevention in countries and regions with heterosexual epidemics, high HIV and low male circumcision prevalence. *Male circumcision provides only partial protection, and therefore should be only one element of a comprehensive HIV prevention package* which includes: the provision of HIV testing and counseling services; treatment for sexually transmitted infections; the promotion of safer sex practices; the provision of male and female condoms and promotion of their correct and consistent use (www.who.int/HIV/topics/malecircumcision/en, accessed 20.7.2015, italics mine).

[110] Ibid. p. 2. - He refers to: Melanie Newman, "Analysis: Circumcision Debated as African Campaign Expands", www.thebureauinvestigates.com. accessed on 29-9-12 [Alufandika]; www.circinfo.org. accessed on 29-9-12 [Alufandika], "Flawed African Circumcision Trials Cannot be Used to Inform U.S. Circumcision Debate." http://www.intactAmerica.org. accessed on 19-12-12 [Alufandika]; *Doctors opposing circumcision HIV statement*, http://www.doctors-opposingcircumcision.org, accessed on 14-4-13 [Alufandika] – I can not assess the truth of either claims independently.

7.2.1 VMMCC as an additional method of reducing HIV transmission

Here I conclude that such a big campaign, to circumcise millions in Africa, was not recommended to improve the protection rate by 1.2% points. The only reason I can see to recommend it was to protect those who practice sex unprotected by condoms. To protect them would be a good moral reason for it. On the other hand, if VMMCC measurably reduces the use of condoms, this moral end is defeated and the campaign which was to reduce the infection rate is actively increasing it.

7.2.2 Statistical evidence

It is reported that in the field trials 5411 circumcised men and 5497 that were uncircumcised took part. After less than two years 1.18%[111] of the circumcised had become HIV positive compared to 2.49%[112] of the uncircumcised.[113] These figures have been questioned as 703 men dropped out of the trials and because of possible bias among the organizers of the trials. It is also claimed that the early termination of the trials was made because the infection rates among circumcised men were comparatively rising.[114] I can not assess these claims with any authority, but whatever the randomized field trials (of 5411-703 men) yielded is open to the much bigger randomized field trial of reality, not over less than two years but over a generation, since HIV came onto the scene. Alufandika reports that in the Muslim provinces of North Eastern Kenya the HIV prevalence is rising,[115] and infection rates of Muslim

---

[111] These infections took place though condoms were recommended and provided free.

[112] These infections took place though condoms were recommended and provided free.

[113] The trials were broken off prematurely, and circumcision was offered to all. (Joseph Alufandika, The Voluntary Male Medical Circumcision (VMMCC) Campaign: Dissemination and Impact. A Case Study of T/A Mbenje in Nsanje, Southern Malawi, BA, Mzuzu University, 2013, p. 8).

[114] Alufandika, p. 8. – I have no way of independently assessing these claims and counter-claims.

[115] *"Soaring Incidence of AIDS among Circumcised Populations … shows that Foreskin not the Problem and Circumcision not the Answer."*

African men in the UK are in no way better than among uncircumcised African men there.[116]

What seems to be true elsewhere, definitely applies to Malawi. In Malawi about 80% of the Yawo are Muslims, and among them all men are circumcised,[117] and for other Muslims circumcision is equally required. This creates a field trial of about 500,000 circumcised men against a control group of maybe 5,000,000 uncircumcised men.[118] In Malawi we do not have HIV infection statistics that separate by religion, tribe or circumcision, but it is clear that the Muslim population dominates some districts in the east like Mangochi and Balaka, and it is also clear that in such districts the infection rates are measurably higher than in the predominantly "Christian" districts.

When presented with this evidence, Dr Mary Kwataine, at that time responsible for the campaign, responded that almost all those Yawo were circumcised in the bush, not under proper hygienic conditions in a hospital (or in temporary medical facilities as the VMMCC provides them). As if this was not enough to prove her point, she added that, after all, in many cases of "bush circumcision" the foreskin is not fully removed, thus making the operation useless in reducing the chance of transmission. She gave no evidence for partial circumcision among the Yawo, nor could she refer to any randomized field trial that measured the different infection rates for partially and fully circumcised men.[119]

I could find no evidence for partial circumcision among the Yawo.[120] The one report available to me shows that care is taken that the whole foreskin is removed, and if, by mistake, something had been left, a

---

[116] Alufandika, p. 19/20.

[117] Circumcision is also widespread among non-Muslim Yawo.

[118] These figures include children and are very rough calculations. But they show the proportions. And even if the circumcised men were only 250,000, that would be much more than in the three randomized field trials that provided the "evidence" for the VMMCC.

[119] Alufandika (p. 19) points out that in the last two Malawi Health Surveys (15-49 years) the infection rate was lower among uncircumcised men (2010: 10% against 8%; 2004: 13.2% against 9.5%). *Malawi 2010 Demographic and Health Survey,* National Statistical Office, Zomba.

[120] This should be checked by Yawo informants. Does the penis after circumcision have any space to collect the smedge which is found normally under the foreskin?

second operation is performed to clean up.[121] I also could not find anything on partial circumcision among the Yawo in Ian Dick's monograph.[122] Different from the Yawo there is evidence for partial circumcision among the Lhomwe,[123] and I have even one report from a Lhomwe initiation camp where the boys were circumcised by *seeing* the knife.[124] But Lomwe practice does not count for the statistics I have presented, as they are only for Yawo and Muslims.[125] Thus, while all statistical evidence is against the claim that circumcision offers protection, the VMMCC sternly adheres to its position.

7.4 The effects on women

The randomized trials were only concerned with HIV transmission from women to men, and they found that such transmission to circumcised men was, though reduced by "up to 60%" still a reality, so that circumcised men would get infected, who could then infect those uninfected female partners they have sex with. Since the penis is much

---

[121] This is an extract from a survey conducted about 20 years ago by a Chancellor College lecturer and his team about Yawo initiation on behalf of the Muslim Association in Malawi: "The Ngaliba pulls out a small piece of wood called 'Kalamu' and a small but very sharp knife or razor blade. The Ngaliba takes the boy's penis in his hands. He inserts the piece of wood called 'Kalamu' inside the foreskin. He then pulls the foreskin above the piece of wood leaving the shaft of the penis behind. This done, he swiftly cuts the foreskin as fast as possible."

[122] Ian Dicks, *An African Worldview. The Muslim Amacinga Yawo of Southern Malaŵi*, Zomba: Kachere, 2012, p. 134.

[123] This is *zoma la aphale* in the *Chidototo* initiation rite. Alufandika (p. 18) points out that for the Yawo and all Muslims circumcision is complete, only among the non-Muslim Lhomwe there is the rite of *Chidototo* which has partial circumcision. In an essay about boys' circumcision among the Lhomwe there is no mention of how much of the prepuce is cut: Francis Bonongwe, "Initiation Rites for Boys in Lomwe Society: A Dying Cultural Practice" in: J.C. Chakanza (ed), *Initiation Rites for Boys in Lomwe Society in Malawi and other Essays*, Zomba: Kachere, 2005, pp. 9-39.

[124] Patrick Makondesa, Christian Initiation Rites in Southern Malawi, Postgraduate Colloquium Presentation, Department of Theology and Religious Studies, University of Malawi, 1999.

[125] There are few Muslims among the Lhomwe.

harder, it causes frequent bruises in the vagina walls, and that facilitates the passage of the virus to the woman.[126]

7.5 The invisible condom or: The listener decides on the meaning of a message

One of my students, in a research on religious change, appropriately included circumcision. He wrote:

> However, it should be noted that the current introduction of voluntary male circumcision by the government poses a great challenge, particularly for the youth in the area. Two boys, my relatives, who are residents of Kombo Village, are said to have caught the pandemic when they tried to have plain sex shortly after undergoing voluntary male circumcision at Lozi Health Centre. When I asked them they revealed to me that, since the government is administering voluntary male circumcision promising 60% protection against HIV/Aids contraction, they decided to benefit from the exercise. Soon after that they decided to taste unprotected sex to see how it feels because they never did it before for fear of contracting HIV/Aids. Now, in order to prove that they were safe, they thought of going for HIV testing, the results of which were found to be positive.[127]

---

[126] Alufandika quotes this outcry: "Why do they claim to be so intent on saving lives by coaxing men to be circumcised yet they are also **so much ignoring how lives of innocent women (plus their unborn children) are being ruined by HIV positive circumcised men?**"

[127] Kaliton Mbuma, The Muslim-Christian Relationships at Kombo Village in Nkhotakota District Central Malawi, BA, Mzuzu University, 2013. He continues his text by referring to the research of one of his colleagues: "Besides, Edward Jeffrey claims that, having heard that *jando* which is practiced among the Yao of Kasamba can reduce HIV infection to 50%, he literally went there to ascertain if at all that was right. According to him, the results indicated that it was not that true because, having been interviewed, one of the initiates, who is now HIV positive, regretted having been misled by such evidently baseless speculations (Edward Jeffrey, The Impact of Jando Initiation on its Initiates in the Area of Kasamba Village in Nkhotakota, BA Mzuzu University, 2012). In a nutshell, this serves to prove beyond doubt that regardless of what is said, circumcision of any kind, be it *jando* which is conducted by a *ngaliba* or the Voluntary Medical Male Circumcision (VMMC) which is administered by government, can be dangerous to health in the case of plain sex.

This is a blatant case where the prevention message, claiming that VMMCC should be taken as an *additional* precaution, was interpreted as offering a replacement for condoms, so it is not ABCD as argued by the campaigners, but ABD, leaving out the highly effective C, which offers up to 98% protection compared to D, which offers 60% protection at best (if we can believe those who proclaim the message.)[128]

Of course, WHO and all other service providers argue that the message ("additional protection") was misunderstood or misinterpreted. This is another false truth, as we all know from communications theory that the listener decides on the meaning of a message, not the sender. And if one and the same message is continuously misunderstood and/or misinterpreted, it is the moral responsibility of the sender to stop the message from being sent. If the "true" message is consistently misunderstood, the moral responsibility for that falls on the sender. I have not come across any study (let alone a randomized field trial) to ascertain how the VMMCC prevention message is understood and applied. Therefore it is irresponsible "to roll out" VMMCC for 80% of all males in Malawi without any (scientific or simple) check on the effects of the millions of Dollars spent on the project.

To repeat: If the VMMCC campaign achieves the opposite of what it claims to promote, it is in itself immoral to continue with it. **WHO does not proclaim that circumcision is the invisible condom, but if many listeners take that to be the message, then WHO (and all who promote VMMC are morally responsible for it.**[129]

7.5.1 A student's findings

For the above argument I have only used three cases of anecdotal evidence. In this section I present the findings of my student, who investigated the effects of VMMCC in Southern Malawi.[130] He found that

---

[128] The three men here described did not take long to get infected, and they show no evidence of less or more protection for *medical* circumcision. Of course, these are only three cases, but the evidence is piling up that they are not atypical.

[129] Leaving aside moral responsibility, does WHO or the Malawian government want that the well intended campaign achieves the opposite?

[130] Joseph Alufandika, The Voluntary Male Medical Circumcision (VMMCC) Campaign: Dissemination and Impact. A Case Study of T/A Mbenje in Nsanje, Southern Malawi, BA, Mzuzu University, 2013. - His sample consisted of 147

out of the men, 79.6% were in favour of circumcision, and 10.9% indicated that "once circumcised they would abandon the other HIV risk-reduction strategies (ABC)."[131]

Of the 33 women interviewed, 31 were in favour of male circumcision as "giving them hope that they could not get infected once they sleep with infected men."[132] Five of the women explicitly confirmed that they would be happy to have unprotected sex with a circumcised man, fearing only pregnancy.[133]

From his observations Alufandika lists these negative effects:

> 1. An increase in promiscuity "induced by the high hopes of immunity said to be offered by circumcision as claimed by the Ministry of Health."[134]
>
> 2. The message of "up to 60% protection" is regularly understood to mean "100% immunity."[135]
>
> 3. There is a reduction in the women's bargaining power for condom usage. (This is a belief for both sexes: the men claim to be immune and women believe that.)
>
> 4. For a woman the circumcised penis has a higher potency of causing bruises in the walls of the vagina and therefore increases the risk of infection.

---

men and 30 women from the 9 Group Village Headmen in the T/A Mbenje area (p. 12-13).

[131] Ibid, p. 13.

[132] Ibid.

[133] Ibid. (Pregnancy can easily be prevented by injections etc these days, condoms are not needed.)

[134] This he supports by reference to Danielle Frisbie (1.10.2012), "Believing Circumcision Prevents HIV, Malawi Men go on 'Sex Spree,'" www.aidscic.org, accessed 26.4.2013 [Joseph Alufandika]. She reports that "74% of circumcised men in Mangochi say that they no longer use condoms and 58% of female sex workers ... say that they do not require their male partners to use condoms once found to be circumcised, and circumcised men also pay less for sex." (I remember similar articles in various issues of the *Nation*).

[135] Alufandika, p. 19, 22. There are several observations that support his observation.

5. There is increased infection rate as the VMMCC offers freely circumcision to all men without ever checking whether they are HIV positive. (And since such men are judged as protected by many women, they spread the infection freely.)[136]

6. The decrease in condom use will lead to an increase in unwanted pregnancies. (He has no such case in his sample, but the logic is clear as not all women who forego condom use will replace the condom by other birth control measures, though they are easily available.)

7.6 Religious Reactions

I have found little information on reactions to the VMMCC from the side of the Christian churches or the Muslim community. Below is what I have found.

7.6.1 Malawi Interfaith Association

I found a leaflet in a medical institution in Mzuzu, showing the pictures of a Catholic Bishop, a Protestant pastor and a Muslim sheik, asking everyone to "help to reduce HIV by encouraging voluntary medical male circumcision (VMMCC) Today." The leaflet argues that "a circumcised man is up to 60% less likely to get HIV than an uncircumcised man!" and that "reduction of HIV prevalence among men means fewer infected [infections] to transit to women." The next paragraph indicates that VMMCC is not enough.[137] I was also shocked to see a crude graph on the relationship between HIV prevalence and MC (Medical Circumcision).[138]

---

[136] This is against the "UNAIDS recommendation which states that the HIV-positive must bring their wives for couple counselling before proceeding with the circumcision" (Alufandika p. 16). The author reports no incidences of such counselling or even HIV testing.

[137] "Within marriage, both partners must know their HIV status and both must remain faithful to each other or use protection. Others may need to be encouraged to reduce the number of sexual partners and to use protection." – This is as confused as the official statements on the issue.

[138] It shows that seven African countries with an HIV prevalence rate between 14.2% and 25.8% have an MC prevalence of below 20% (Mozambique, Swaziland, Zambia, Namibia, Botswana and Zimbabwe in ascending order) and that 11 countries between 12.8% and 2.1% (Rwanda, Kenya, Congo, Cameroon, Nigeria, Gabon, Liberia, Sierra Leone, Ghana, Benin and Guinea, in descending order) have an MC prevalence of over 80%. Maybe I am not properly trained in

7.6.2 Adventist Development Relief Agency (ADRA)

I have no official statement from the Seventh-day Adventist Church in Malawi, but ADRA director Michael Usi, at a news conference on 14.8.2015 in Blantyre, warned of an "unprecedented new wave of HIV infections in the country if campaign messages on circumcision are not disseminated correctly."[139] He argued that:

> 1. Despite the emphasis by the campaigners that circumcision only reduces the risk of contracting the virus, the information management on the subject is poor.
>
> 2. The campaigners do not tell one when to have sex after circumcision.
>
> 3. "A lot of men are excited with circumcision and indulge in unprotected sex immediately the wound heals, believing they are safe."
>
> 4. "Circumcision campaigners have failed to encourage people to continue abstaining, remain faithful or use a condom."
>
> 5. "They do not bother to ask you if you are HIV positive or not."[140]
>
> 6. "It is regrettable that women have been completely left out of the campaign."[141]

I have no information from other churches or from any of the groups of the Muslim community.

7.7 The Morality of the Voluntary Male Medical Circumcision Campaign

How moral is the Voluntary Male Medical Circumcision Campaign? The answer is simple: The only thing that can be called "moral" are the good

---

reading such statistics, but I can not believe that in Africa there are no countries that have an MC prevalence rate of between 20 and 79%. Or have these countries been excluded deliberately? And if so, why?

[139] Frank Namangale, "Circumcision Campaign Worries ADRA," *The Nation*, 15.8.2014, p. 4.

[140] Alufandika observed the same problem, which is, of course, against the rules, but obviously a reality.

[141] Michael Usi demands that women should be explicitly warned of the dangers of having unprotected sex with circumcised men.

intentions, while the consequences are immoral, and the blame must not be put on "those who misinterpret the message," but on those authorities that send out the message without checking on the effects.

8. Conclusion

I understand the quest of people for healing. I do understand that at the time of Chisupe, when there was no healing for HIV/AIDS on any level, desperate or hopeful people would try anything that became available. I do not understand that people now, when ARVs are easily available and proven successful, prefer healing procedures (herbs, prayers or a mixture of both) that have no evidence in their favour. It is a pity that God's name is continually misused by those who claim to serve him, and that instead of healing in too many cases death has resulted. And equally I do not understand how a multi-million Dollar campaign to save lives can clearly defeat its own end and still be maintained.

Bibliography

Unpublished

Alufandika, Joseph, The Voluntary Male Medical Circumcision (VMMCC) Campaign: Dissemination and Impact. A Case Study of T/A Mbenje in Nsanje, Southern Malawi, BA, Mzuzu University, 2013.

Banda, Khetwayo, Word Alive Ministries International (WAMI) and its Wholistic Mission, MA, Mzuzu University, 2012.

Chirwa, Frank, Theology of Health in the Seventh-day Adventist Church: A Quest for Abundant Life in Jesus, Mzuni Documents no. 112, 2010.

Jeffrey, Edward, The Impact of Jando Initiation on its Initiates in the Area of Kasamba Village in Nkhotakota, BA, Mzuzu University, 2012.

Makondesa, Patrick, Christian Initiation Rites in Southern Malawi, Postgraduate Colloquium Presentation, Department of Theology and Religious Studies, University of Malawi, 1999.

Malisa, Nahori, Analyzing Critical HIV and AIDS Results in Malawi. A Case Study of an Interface between Christian Faith/Traditional Healing Claims and Scientific Treatment, BA, Mzuzu University.

Manda, Bridget, Women and Witchcraft Accusations: A Case of Zomba Urban, MA Module, Mzuzu University, 2011.

Mbuma, Kaliton, The Muslim-Christian Relationships at Kombo Village in Nkhotakota District Central Malawi, BA, Mzuzu University, 2013.

Published

Bonongwe, Francis, "Initiation Rites for Boys in Lomwe Society: A Dying Cultural Practice" in: J.C. Chakanza (ed), *Initiation Rites for Boys in Lomwe Society in Malawi and other Essays*, Zomba: Kachere, 2005, pp. 9-39.

Choy, Leona, *Andrew Murray. Apostle of Abiding Love*, Ft Washington: CLC, 1978.

DeGabriele, Joe, *Chisupe, Old Peppers don't Bite*, Zomba: Kachere, 1996.

DeGabriele, Joseph, "When Pills don't Work – African Illnesses, Misfortune and Mdulo," *Religion in Malawi*, No. 9, 1999, pp. 9-23

Dicks, Ian, *An African Worldview. The Muslim Amacinga Yawo of Southern Malaŵi*, Zomba: Kachere, 2012.

Doran, Marissa, "Reconstructing Mchape '95: AIDS, Billy Chisupe, and the Politics of Persuasion," *Journal of Eastern African Studies*, 1:3, pp 397-416, published online 10.10.2007.

du Plessis, J., *The Life of Andrew Murray of South Africa,* London/Edinburgh/New York, 1919.

Dzanja, Langford L., *Chipatala cha Chilengedwe. Machiritso Kupyolera mu Chilengedwe.* 1, np: Advent Publications, nd [2014].

Fiedler, Klaus, "Compulsory HIV Testing. A Christian Imperative," *Religion in Malawi* no. 14, 2007, pp. 33-39.

Fiedler, Klaus, "'We are all Infected or Affected' - The Moralities of Antiretroviral Treatment", *Journal of Humanities,* no. 18 (2004), pp 19-37.

Fiedler, Klaus, "Access to ARVs and the Role of the Churches," *Religion in Malawi,* no. 12, 2005, pp. 6-10; "The Moralities of Condom Use. Theological Considerations," *Religion in Malawi* 2006, pp. 32-37;

Fiedler, Klaus, *Conflicted Power in Malawian Christianity. Essays Missionary and Evangelical from Malawi,* Mzuzu: Mzuni Press, 2015.

Fiedler, Klaus, *Ganz auf Vertrauen. Geschichte und Kirchenverständnis der Glaubensmissionen,* Gießen/Basel, Brunnen Verlag, 1992; out of print, but available on http://tinyurl.com/fiedler for free download.

Fiedler, Rachel NyaGondwe, *Coming of Age. A Christianized Initiation among Women in Southern Malawi,* Zomba: Kachere, 2005.

Makondesa, Patrick, *The Church History of Providence Industrial Mission 1900-1940,* Zomba: Kachere, 2006.

National Statistical Office, *Malawi 2010 Demographic and Health Survey,* National Statistical Office, Zomba.

Mlenga, Joyce, *Dual Religiosity in Northern Malawi,* Mzuzu: Mzuni Press, 2016.

Murray, Andrew, Divine Healing. A Series of Addresses and Personal Testimony, London: Victory Press, 1900.

Namangale, Frank, "Circumcision Campaign Worries ADRA," *The Nation,* 15.8.2014.

Probst, Peter, "'Mchape' '95, or, the Sudden Fame of Billy Goodson Chisupe: Healing, Social Memory and the Enigma of the Public Sphere in Post-Banda Malawi," *Africa,* Vol. 69, no 1, (1999), pp. 108-137.

Schoffeleers, Matthew, "The AIDS Pandemic, the Prophet Billy Chisupe, and the Democratization Process in Malawi," *Journal of Religion in Africa,* vol 29:4, pp. 406-441.

Sharra, Albert, "Probing HIV Cure Herbs: Who is Losing?" *Weekend Nation,* 7.2.2015, pp. 20-21.

Soko, Boston, *Nchimi Chikanga. The Battle against Witchcraft in Malawi,* Blantyre: CLAIM-Kachere, 2002.

Strohbehn, Ulf, *The Zionist Churches in Malawi - History - Theology - Anthropology*, Mzuzu: Mzuni Press, 2016.

Web

Chiumia, Sintha and Julian Rademeyer, "Claim that Malawi 'wonder herb' cures HIV is untrue and irresponsible" (https://africacheck.org/reports/claim-that-..., published 9.6.2013, accessed 8.10.2016).

Chvyunguma, Tendayi, "Exit Mchape and Chambe, enters Wizika. Malawian Herbalist Claims" (malawi24.com/2015/05/23/exit-mchape-and-chambe-enters-wizika..., accessed 20.7.2015 and 7.10.2016).

Doctors opposing circumcision HIV statement, http://www.doctorsopposingcircumcision.org, accessed on 14-4-13 [Joseph Alufandika]

Frisbie, Danielle, (1.10.2012), "Believing Circumcision Prevents HIV, Malawi Men go on 'Sex Spree,'" www.aidscic.org, accessed 26.4.2013 [Joseph Alufandika].

https://africacheck.org/reports/a-roundup-of-fake-aids-cures-angels-zapper-garani-mw1-topvein-sf-2000/ (accessed 20.10.2016)

Newman, Melanie, "Analysis: Circumcision Debated as African Campaign Expands", www.thebureauinvestigates.com. accessed on 29.9.2012 [Joseph Alufandika];

www.circinfo.org. accessed on 29.9.2012 [Alufandika], "Flawed African Circumcision Trials Cannot be Used to Inform U.S. Circumcision Debate." http://www.intactAmerica.org. accessed 19.12.2012 [Alufandika].

www.dacb.org/stories/ southafrica/murray_jr.html.

www.investigator.co.ug/crime/item/14983-ugandan-born-again...

www.who.int/HIV/topics/malecircumcision /en, accessed 20.7.2015).

www.ingramcontent.com/pod-product-compliance
Lightning Source LLC
Chambersburg PA
CBHW051119230426
43667CB00014B/2649